ALKALINE DIET S

AMAZING ASIAN ALK VEGAN) RECIPES FOR WEIGHT LOSS, VITALITY, AND WELLNESS

By Marta Tuchowska

All information in this book has been carefully researched and checked for factual accuracy. However, the author and publishers make no warranty, expressed or implied, that the information contained herein is appropriate for every individual, situation or purpose, and assume no responsibility for errors or omission. The reader assumes the risk and full responsibility for all actions, and the author will not be held liable for any loss or damage, whether consequential, incidental, and special or otherwise that may result from the information presented in this publication. By purchasing this book you have agreed to the above-mentioned statement.

All cooking is an experiment in a sense, and many people come to the same or similar recipe over time. All recipes in this book have been derived from author's personal experience. Should any bear a close resemblance to those used elsewhere, that is purely coincidental.

The book is not intended to provide medical advice or to take the place of medical advice and treatment from your personal physician. Readers are advised to consult their own doctors or other qualified health professionals regarding the treatment of medical conditions. The author shall not be held liable or responsible for any misunderstanding or misuse of the information contained in this book. The information is not intended to diagnose, treat or cure any disease.

From the Author

Thank you for taking an interest in my book. It really means a lot to me!

Because I am so grateful for you, I would like you to receive all of my upcoming releases for free or only 99c. All you need to do is to join my Alkaline Wellness Newsletter. Don't worry about spam or annoying marketing e-mails. You see, the reason why I have a mailing list, is to connect with my readers. I hate spam as much as you do.

Join my free newsletter at:

www.holisticwellnessproject.com/alkaline

As a welcome gift, you will receive a free copy of my book: "Revolutionize Your Life with Alkaline Foods" + 2 bonus eBooks (yummy desserts included). You will also be receiving many powerful motivational and inspirational reminders with a holistic touch +weekly healthy recipes + insider news+ amazing wellness tips + other recommendations.

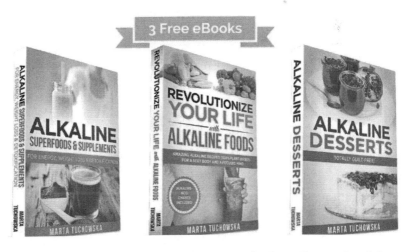

Now, let the journey begin. Are you ready for vibrant health and unstoppable energy?

We have some pretty amazing recipes to try today!

THE ALKALINE DIET SPICED UP

I am a big fan of the alkaline diet and it honestly is a huge part of my lifestyle. I truly believe it is a natural wellness and detoxification tool that can provide us with endless energy levels, focus, zest for life, and even prevent many 21st century diseases (poor digestion, migraines, adrenal exhaustion due to overindulgence in caffeine, etc.). Weight loss comes as a "secondary" effect and there is no need to worry about counting calories on the alkaline diet. Really!

From my own experience, I can tell you that my transition to alkalinity was not simple. Even though I was excited to keep it alkaline, I would lack certain practical tools in the form of new mouth-watering dishes. It was also hard to see my friends and family eating their "regular stuff" while I was drooling over another big bowl of salad. Don't get me wrong, I love salads and I eat them regularly. But let's be real - we all need to give ourselves some eating pleasure and experiment with different tastes, textures and flavors. If our taste buds are happy, we will be more set up for the long-term, healthy lifestyle success.

In all my books you will hear me say that the Alkaline Diet is not just a diet; it is a lifestyle, a holistic lifestyle. This is what I am stressing again. Even if you are following some other diet of your choice, your body and mind will be grateful when you feed them with more alkaline foods (=more fresh veggies and some fruit). For example, give your body alkaline juices, salads, soups, and dips. Alkalinity is compatible with other diets. Even if you are not 100% vegan, you can still benefit by looking for dairy-free and meat-free alternatives. Going alkaline does not mean going vegan (unless you want to), but it does overlap a lot with the vegan lifestyle. Meat and dairy are considered to be acid-forming foods and must be either eliminated or drastically reduced. The recipes included in this book are the best combination of vegan and alkaline lifestyles.

No matter what kind of transition you are scheduling for yourself (I am always very open-minded and respectful about different diets), you need to prepare yourself. Acquiring new, alkaline diet inspired cooking skills should form a part of your plan.

This is what this book will teach you. I wanted to keep it simple and easy - perfect for the modern, busy people in the 21st century.

So how did this book come about? It's simple. When I first got started on the Alkaline Diet, I had many ups and downs and found it difficult to keep on track. I just lacked a plan and would attract failure instead of success. Read more about it in "The Alkaline Satisfaction Cookbook". It wasn't until I committed myself to learning and cooking at least one new, delicious, and exciting alkaline recipe a week that I truly committed to the alkaline lifestyle. I loved the process of alkalizing my body and mind and having fun while doing so.

My boyfriend was a bit reluctant at first. He thought that the alkaline diet was only about salads, green smoothies, weird detoxes, and who knows what. He said it was for rabbits. This is why I became committed to preparing mouthwatering alkaline dishes to get him on my side and I'm happy to say I had success with that. He has acquired many new, healthy, alkaline habits and this lifestyle helped him cure serious digestive problems. Doctors would just prescribe another pill that eventually would reverberate on his general wellness and energy levels. Simple alkaline habits helped him find balance, restore health and easy digestive problems. It worked as a natural medicine.

I then decided to throw regular healthy dinner parties for friends to spark their interest in Alkalinity. They loved my dishes and very often would not believe that this was the "famous rabbit diet". I would explain to them all about the nutritional value, and how you can reduce meat and dairy by adding foods like quinoa, tofu, almond milk, and seaweed. Of course, the trick is to learn how to prepare those foods so that they taste great. My book is a result of my alkaline cooking experiments that I want to share with you. You can set yourself off for alkaline success and improve your overall health and wellness with this diet. You can also transition yourself towards a more environment friendly, vegan inspired lifestyle. If you already are a vegan - congratulations!

Everyone is welcome - vegans, non-vegans, wellness nuts, alkaline diet lovers, alkaline diet beginners, vegetarians, and anyone interested in creative cooking, and a healthy lifestyle.

I invite you to join my amazing alkaline party and discover how much fun and excitement you can bring to your new, healthy, balanced, holistic alkaline lifestyle. Aside from taking care of yourself, you can also take care of your loved ones and the entire world. Going "Alkalarian" is a decision you will never regret.

I nearly forgot to mention that most of my recipes are also gluten free. Since gluten is acid forming, "alkalarians" always try to go for non-gluten options.

I would love to say thanks to all my Indian friends who taught me about a great deal of spices and herbs so that I could infuse my alkaline diet with a myriad of incredible tastes and flavors.

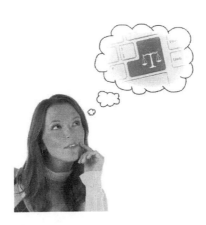

Never heard of the Alkaline Diet and don't know where to start?

I remember when I first learned about the alkaline diet. I was more than confused and skeptical. I wanted to take action but didn't know how. I would spend endless hours online looking for alkaline-acid charts only to find there was way too much contradictory information out there.

I don't want you to feel confused. I also really appreciate the fact you took an interest in my work. This is why I would love to offer you a <u>free, complimentary 100 page e-book</u> and **easy alkaline-acid charts** (printable so that you can keep them on your fridge or in your wallet). It will provide a solid foundation to kick-start your alkaline diet success. You will get all the facts explained in plain English, practical alkaline tips, and yummy, vegan-friendly recipes full of taste, motivational advice, as well as printable charts for quick reference. I will also show you how to combine the alkaline lifestyle with other diets (Paleo, vegetarian, vegan). The alkaline diet is very flexible, and it always welcome all kinds of "Alkalarians." You don't have to be 100% vegan to follow an alkaline diet, the choice is always yours.

The most important thing is to listen to your body. You don't have to follow through 100% the first time if that's not what works for you. For example, there might be some really healthy ingredients and they may be labeled as alkaline, but if your body does not tolerate them, reject them and choose what works for you. We all have unique preferences and tastes - and so when creating a diet that works for us, we need to learn to be selective.

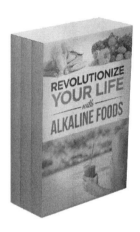

Visit the links below and grab your free copy of <u>Revolutionize Your Life with Foods</u> now, before you forget.

Download link:

www.holisticwellnessproject.com/alkaline

In case you happen to have any problems with your free download, email us at:

info@holisticwellnessproject.com

Recipe Measurements

I love keeping ingredient measurements as simple as possible-this is why I stick to tablespoons, teaspoons and cups.

The cup measurement I use is the American cup measurement. I also use it for dry ingredients. If you are new to it, let me help you:

If you don't have American Cup measures, just use a metric or imperial liquid measuring jug and fill your jug with your ingredient to the corresponding level. Here's how to go about it:

1 American Cup= 250ml= 8 fl.oz

For example:

If a recipe calls for 1 cup of almonds, simply place your almonds into your measuring jug until it reaches the 250 ml/8oz mark.

I know that different countries use different measurements and I wanted to make things simple for you.

Translations (US-UK English)

Eggplant=Aubergine

Zucchini=Courgette

Cilantro=Coriander

Garbanzo Beans=Chickpeas

Navy Beans-=Haricot Beans

Aragula=Rocket

Broth=Stock

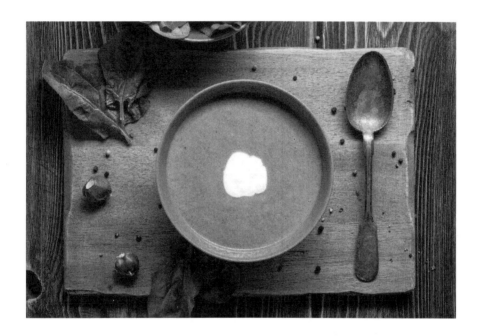

Yellow Mung Bean Curry

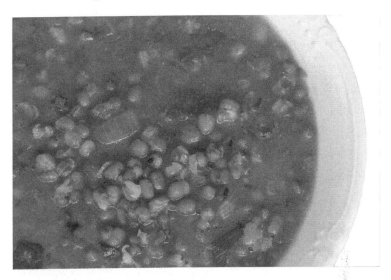

Serves: 3
Ingredients:
- 1 cup mung beans (*rinsed under cool running water*)
- 7-8 spinach leaves
- ¼ teaspoon turmeric powder
- 2 medium tomatoes, chopped
- Half teaspoon Himalaya salt
- coconut oil (1-2 tablespoons)
- 1 teaspoon mustard seeds
- Handful of fresh curry leaves
- 1 teaspoon cumin
- Fresh lemon juice (1-2 tablespoons)
- Asafetida (half teaspoon)
- 2- minced cloves of garlic
- 1 green chili, finely chopped

- 3 cups water

Method
1. Boil the mung beans in the 3 cups of water along with a

pinch of salt until they are tender.

2. Heat some coconut oil in a large sauce pan.

3. Add some mustard seeds, cumin, asafetida, and turmeric. Finally, add the curry leaves. Add chopped chili, tomatoes and sauté them for 7-8 minutes.

4. Add the spinach and mung beans.

5. Add salt, lemon juice and cook for 7-8 minutes with the lid covered.

6. Garnish with chopped coriander and serve along with some whole-wheat bread or brown rice.

7. Enjoy!

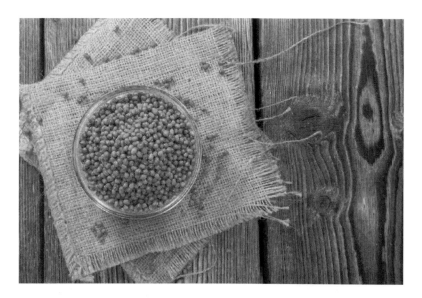

Mung beans are very nutritious and a great source of: Protein, Thiamin, Niacin, Vitamin B6, Pantothenic Acid, Iron, Magnesium, Phosphorus and Potassium, Vitamin C, Vitamin K, Riboflavin, Folate, Copper and Manganese. They blend extremely well with tasty, oriental dishes. I also recommend you try some mung beans sprouts when you get a chance.

Pumpkin Smoothie

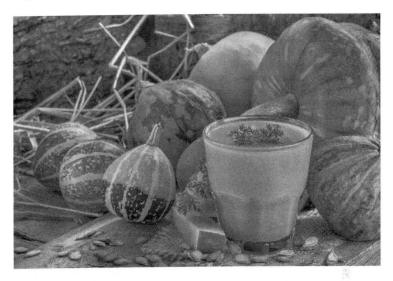

This recipe is a great, quick meal replacement, in case you are pressed for time. Can be served on all occasions, especially as a snack or aperitif.

Serves: 3

Ingredients:

- 1 cup chopped pumpkin (steamed)
- 1 cup coconut milk
- ¼ cup almond milk
- ½ avocado
- ¼ teaspoon cinnamon powder
- ¼ teaspoon all-spice powder
- ¼ teaspoon nutmeg powder
- OPTIONAL: 1 teaspoon vanilla essence
- 1 tablespoon flax seeds
- A few drops of stevia (optional)
- Some ice cubes

Method

1. Blend until smooth.

2. Pour this pumpkin smoothie into a large glass.
3. Add some ice cubes and serve. Enjoy!

All spices and herbs are alkalizing and have anti-inflammatory properties. So even if you have a recipe that is not so alkaline, you can always spice it up by adding some aromatic herbs and spices. Also, don't worry about calorie counting. It's not about eating less calories, it's about eating right. Coconut milk is extremely nutritious and good for you and so is almond milk. There is no need to restrict it or get obsessed about counting calories (let's take care of your emotional wellness). Flax seeds are rich in Magnesium, Phosphorus, Copper as well as dietary fiber and I really recommend you add them into your diet (they are great for smoothies, cakes, desserts and as a snack).

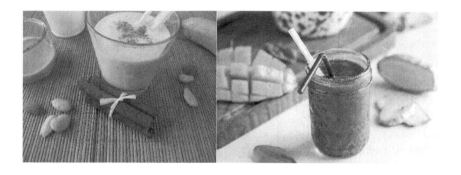

Alkaline Vegan Salad

The Alkaline Lifestyle encourages you to add more raw foods into your diet. Salads are a great and simple way to achieve it and they are easy and quick to prepare. They are the perfect solution for busy people! I love apples in my salads - so refreshing.

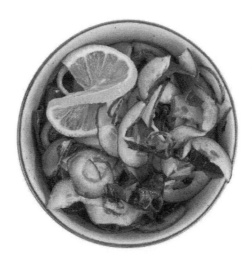

Serves: 3
Ingredients:
- 1 cup chopped apples (optional)
- 1 cup cucumber, (peeled and sliced)
- 1 cup pomegranate seeds (optional)
- 1 jalapeño chili
- 1 medium onion (peeled and chopped)
- 10-15 raw almonds
- 1 minced garlic clove
- 1 tablespoon lemon juice
- ½ teaspoon lemon zest
- Half teaspoon of pepper powder

- 2 tablespoons raisins
- 7-8 lettuce leaves
- ½ teaspoon Himalaya salt
- 1 tablespoon olive oil
- A few square inches of wakame seaweed, previously soaked in water as per instructions

Method

1. Combine all the ingredients in a big bowl, starting with all the veggies, then the fruits, wakame and spices. Garlic, onions and raisins make an interesting combination which I personally love, but I know that not everyone does...try it! You can create different layers, or arrange the salad the way you like.
2. Drizzle some olive oil on top and toss well. Add salt to taste.
3. Serve immediately or refrigerate for 2 hours.
4. It's better served cold. Enjoy!

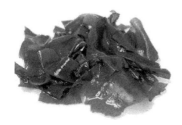

I know that wakame seaweed may seem strange at first, but don't reject it before you have even tried it. It's a really powerful superfood and it is very affordable. It's also easy to store and great for salads, soups and even smoothies. It will energize your body and mind with Riboflavin, Folate, Calcium, Iron, Magnesium, Copper and Manganese – the perfect combination for active lifestyles. And...despite the common belief ("OMG! It's a rabbit diet!"), salads can be extremely nutritious!

Alkaline Green Shake

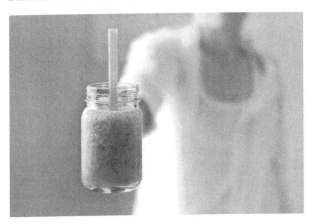

Serves: 2
Ingredients:

- 10-12 spinach leaves
- 1 avocado
- 1 peeled and sliced cucumber
- ½ cup of parsley
- ½ cup of cherry tomatoes
- Some chopped celery
- Some chopped cilantro
- ½ teaspoon Himalaya salt
- Pinch of curry
- 1 cup of water
- 1 cup of almond milk or coconut milk

Method

1. Blend all the ingredients along with some water until smooth consistency is achieved. Ensure that there is no lump formation. If you want a thinner mixture add some more water and blend again.

2. Optional: add some thick coconut milk/coconut cream

17

on top. I also like to add a couple of teaspoons of good quality organic green powder (for example powdered alfalfa).

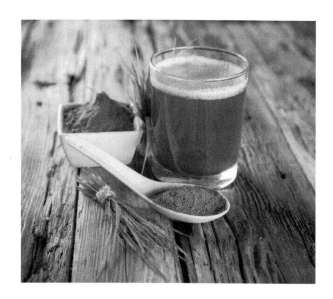

Alfalfa powder will provide you with protein and many vitamins like vitamins A, B1, B6, C, E, and K. Add to it calcium, iron and zinc. Cheers to your health; enjoy!

Super Healthy Alkaline Wraps

Mushrooms are not considered alkaline, but they are still healthy and OK in your 20-30% diet. The alkaline diet is not about eating 100% alkaline. Balance is the key. Be sure to download your food lists + free recipe eBook at: www.HolisticWellnessProject.com/alkaline

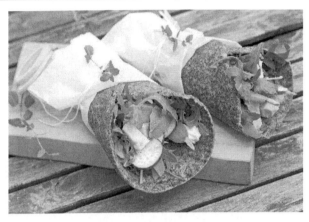

Serves: 3
Ingredients:
- ½ cup chopped mushrooms
- A few radishes, sliced
- A few carrot slices
- 1 sliced sweet onion
- ½ cup dill leaves or/and cilantro
- 1 teaspoon garlic powder
- 1 tablespoon olive oil
- 1 tablespoon apple cider vinegar
- ½ teaspoon salt
- ½ teaspoon cayenne pepper
- 1 chopped avocado
- teaspoon organic barbecue sauce

- 3 gluten-free tortilla wraps

Method

1. Heat some oil in a sauce pan. Sauté the chopped onion until it turns slightly brownish.
2. Throw in the bell peppers, avocado, chopped mushrooms and sauté for another 3-4 minutes until they become tender.
3. Add dill leaves, garlic powder, apple cider vinegar, cayenne pepper, salt and barbecue sauce.
4. Cook for 2-3 minutes. Now switch off the flame.
5. Fill this mixture in each of the wraps.
6. Enjoy!

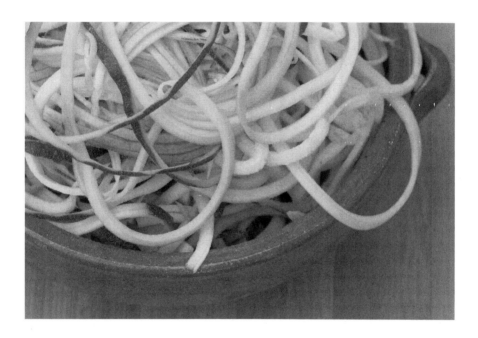

Yummy Veggie Quinoa Soup

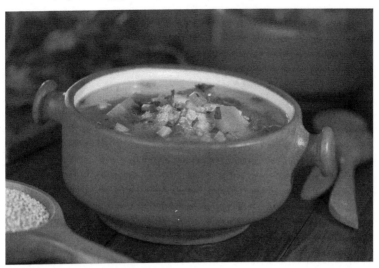

Serves: 2
Ingredients:

- 1 cup quinoa
- 1 ½ tablespoon organic bouillon powder
- 1 cup water
- 1 cup broccoli florets
- 1-2 carrots
- ½ cup chopped leeks
- 1 tablespoon lime juice
- ¼ cup dill leaves
- 1 teaspoon Bragg Liquid Aminos (or soy sauce – soy sauce is not alkaline, but is okay to consume in small amounts)
- Some cilantro
- ½ teaspoon salt
- ½ teaspoon cayenne pepper

Method

1. Boil a cup of water (use a large saucepan) Add the bouillon powder, quinoa and cook for about 15-16

minutes without the lid. Once the quinoa turns nice and fluffy, switch off the flame. You can add some more water if it gets absorbed by the quinoa prior to being fully cooked.

2. Take some water in another saucepan, bring it to a boil and add the leeks, carrots, broccoli, and the lime juice.
3. As soon as the broccoli is tenderized, add the quinoa mixture to this saucepan along with some salt, cayenne pepper, and soy sauce and give it a stir.
4. Let it simmer for about 4-5 minutes.
5. Use some fresh cilantro leaves to garnish. It will also give your dish an incredible oriental taste. Enjoy!

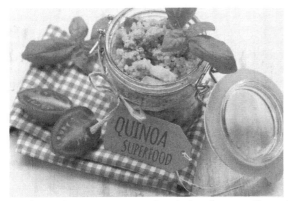

Quinoa is a super grain, it is gluten-free (yes!) and a fantastic source of Magnesium, Phosphorus, and Manganese. To learn more about it (I am kind of addicted to it) check out my article:
www.holisticwellnessproject.com/blog/health-wellness/health-benefits-of-quinoa

Vegan Alkaline Pasta

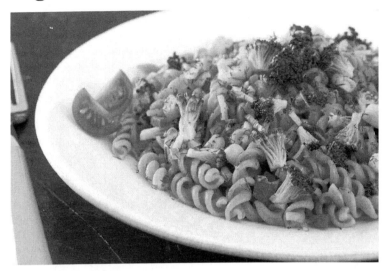

This is my winter comfort food! Perfect for family and friends' dinners and long, cold evenings.

Serves: 2

Ingredients:

- 2 thinly sliced carrots
- 1 thinly sliced zucchini or sliced into strips
- 2 thinly sliced squash
- 1 diced bell pepper
- 1 onion (diced)
- ½ cup broccoli florets
- ¼ cup pasta sauce (I suggest you make your own - simply blend a couple of tomatoes with garlic and olive oil)
- 2 tablespoons olive oil
- 2 tablespoons Italian seasoning
- 1 tablespoon dried basil
- ½ cup chopped tomatoes
- 1 cup gluten-free (or other of your choice) pasta

(boiled). You can also use spelt pasta (not gluten-free though)
- Half teaspoon salt
- Half teaspoon black pepper

Method
OPTION 1:
1. In a bowl, mix all the veggies - carrots, zucchini, bell pepper, and broccoli along with salt, some pepper, and a dash of olive oil and toss well.
2. Lay out this mixture on a baking tray and bake it for about 20 minutes until they turn slightly brownish.
3. Once done, toss the veggies along with some pasta, Italian seasoning and dried basil. Add a bit of pasta sauce.
4. In another baking tray, lay down the squash pieces at the bottom and layer it with the pasta mixture. Repeat this process a couple of times if you want more layers.
5. Bake the pasta in a preheated oven for about 30-35 minutes at 350 degrees Fahrenheit. (or 180 Celsius). Mix well.
6. Enjoy!

OPTION 2:
1. Cook the pasta as per instructions.
2. Stir-fry all the veggies except tomatoes in some coconut oil (low heat).
3. Mix pasta with the veggies, add tomatoes and the seasoning.
4. Enjoy!

Winter Special Leafy Veggie Curry

Do you need to warm up and replenish your energy? Try this recipe. It's also a great naturally healing meal for those suffering from winter colds and flu.

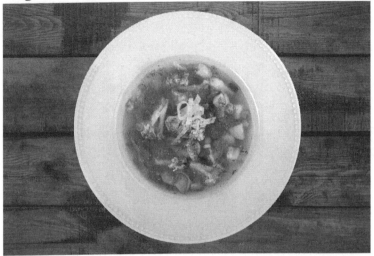

Serves: 3
Ingredients:

- 1 cup mustard leaves
- 1 cup spinach (blanched)
- 1 chopped green chili
- 3 minced garlic cloves
- 1 teaspoon minced ginger
- ¼ teaspoon turmeric powder
- 2 finely chopped onions
- 2 chopped tomatoes
- 3 tablespoon chickpea flour
- 1 cup water
- 1-2 tablespoons of coconut oil
- 1-2 teaspoons of mustard seeds
- ½ teaspoon cumin

- ½ teaspoon Himalaya salt

Optional: 1 teaspoon stevia or maple syrup

Method:

1. Take some water in a saucepan and throw in the mustard leaves, blanched spinach, ginger, chopped chili and cook it on a low flame for 20 minutes.
2. Once all the green veggies are cooked, blend them in a food processor until smooth.
3. Heat some coconut oil in another sauce pan. Add the mustard seeds, cumin and let it crackle followed by turmeric powder.
4. Add the chopped onions, tomatoes and sauté them for about 7-8 minutes.
5. Now add the green veggie paste to the saucepan and cook for 5 minutes.
6. Lastly add the chickpea flour, salt, stevia (or maple syrup) and cook for a few more minutes while continuously stirring the mixture.
7. This dish is best served with gluten-free rice cakes/bread/wraps.

Shitake Rice

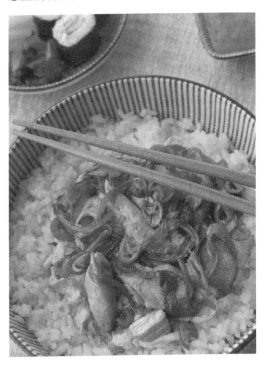

Serves: 3
Ingredients:

- 1 cup brown rice, soaked in water for 8-10 hours
- 1 cup sliced shitake mushrooms (or other mushrooms of your choice- mushrooms are considered acidic, but we can make an exception here, the alkaline diet is not about eating only 100% alkaline foods - it's about maintaining balance.)
- ½ cup green peas
- 1 thinly chopped carrot
- 1 thinly chopped bell pepper
- 3 minced garlic cloves
- 1 teaspoon minced ginger
- 2 sliced sweet onions

27

- 1 tablespoon coconut oil
- 1 ½ tablespoon soy sauce
- 1 teaspoon cane sugar
- ¾ teaspoon salt
- 2 cups water
- 1 slit green chili
- Some cilantro leaves

Method:

1. Take some water in a sauce pan and bring it to a boil. Throw in the brown rice and cook for about 30 minutes. Drain the water, set it aside.
2. Heat some coconut oil in a sauce pan. Add minced garlic, onions, green chili and sauté for about 2-3 minutes. Slide in the minced ginger, mushrooms, chopped carrots, green peas, bell pepper, soy sauce and sauté again until the veggies turn tender.
3. Add the cooked brown rice, salt, cane sugar and fry for 3-4 minutes.
4. Garnish with some cilantro leaves and serve hot.

Vegetable Momos

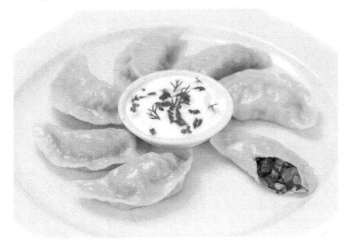

I love this Indian recipe! It combines great taste and nutrition.

Serves: 2-4

Ingredients:

- 1 finely chopped large onion
- 1 finely chopped bell pepper
- 4 carrots (finely chopped)
- 1 cup thinly shredded cabbage
- 1 jalapeno chili
- 1 teaspoon garlic powder
- Some chopped coriander
- 1 cup of mixed sprouts (soy, alfalfa)
- 1 tablespoon soy sauce (optional)
- ¼ teaspoon pepper
- ½ teaspoon salt for the filling + ¼ teaspoon for the dough
- 1 cup chickpea flower
- 2 tablespoons olive oil
- Some water for the dough

Method:

1. Heat some oil in a sauce pan and sauté the onions along with bell peppers, carrots, shredded cabbage and sprouts for about 5-6 minutes.
2. Add some salt, chopped jalapeno chili, soy sauce, pepper, and toss well. Set aside.
3. Knead slightly firm dough using some chickpea flour, salt and water.
4. Roll the dough. Shape it into small circles.
5. Fill in the momo mixture one by one into these rolls and fold them gently.
6. Place the momos in a steamer and cook for about 12-15 minutes.
7. Serve them along with some soy sauce (not really alkaline), or with herb and garlic infused olive oil (super alkaline). It's up to you which option you choose!

Tofu in Mint Sauce

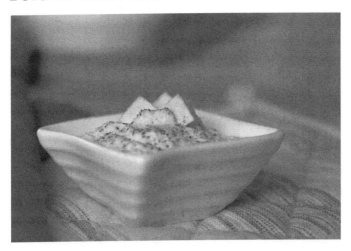

This recipe is extremely refreshing and alkaline! Make sure you choose good quality tofu though.

Serves: 4
Ingredients:

- 1 cup diced tofu
- ½ cup fresh mint leaves
- ½ cup coriander leaves
- 1 green chili
- 1 tablespoon lemon juice
- Pinch of Himalaya salt
- ½ teaspoon pepper
- 1 diced green bell pepper
- 1 diced red bell pepper
- 2 diced onions
- 1 cup cubed pineapple
- 1 tablespoon organic barbecue sauce
- ½ tablespoon oregano
- ½ teaspoon basil (dried)

- 2 tablespoons olive oil (or coconut oil)
- 3-4 skewers

Method:

1. Make a smooth paste of chopped mint, coriander, lemon juice, green chili and salt using a blender.
2. Coat the diced tofu in the mint sauce and set it aside for 60 minutes.
3. Heat some oil in a sauce pan. Sauté the onions and bell peppers for about 2-3 minutes. Switch off the flame.
4. Insert the diced onions, bell pepper, pineapple and marinated tofu onto a skewer.
5. Sprinkle some dried basil and oregano on it.
6. Heat some oil in a sauce pan and fry them for about 5-6 minutes on each side until they turn slightly brown.
7. Serve hot.

Asian Style Noodle Salad

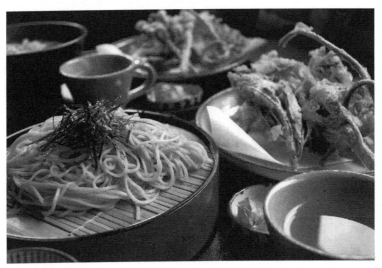

Serves: 3
Ingredients:

- 1 cup shitake or button mushrooms, chopped
- ½ cup chopped and blanched kale leaves
- ½ cup blanched broccoli florets
- 1 medium onion, sliced
- 2 tablespoons of olive oil
- ¾ teaspoon pepper
- ½ teaspoon salt
- ½ cup sprouts
- 1 teaspoon dark soy sauce (low sodium)
- 1 cup soba noodles
- About 2 cups water to boil the noodles
- Some chopped parsley for garnish

Method:

1. Take some water in a large sauce pan and bring it to a boil. Add half a teaspoon of olive oil so the noodles don't stick to each other.

2. Slide in the noodles and cook for about 3-4 minutes until they become slightly tender. Remember not to overcook the noodles. Drain the water. Set aside.

3. Take a salad bowl and mix the mushrooms along with kale leaves, broccoli florets, onion, noodles, pepper, salt, soy sauce and sprouts.

4. Drizzle some olive oil on top and toss.

5. Garnish with chopped parsley. Enjoy!

Spanish Gazpacho Made Oriental

You have probably tried the traditional Spanish gazpacho which is like a tomato and cucumber smoothie with olives, olive oil, vinegar and garlic. Well, I have made it more oriental, spicy and super alkaline...

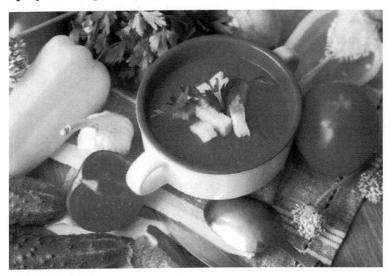

Serves: 2
Ingredients:
- 6 tomatoes (I suggest you remove the peel)
- 4 cucumbers
- ½ tablespoon curry powder
- 1 tablespoon cilantro
- ¼ cup coconut milk
- 2 tablespoons of coconut oil
- Juice of 2 limes
- 2 garlic cloves
- Pinch of chilli powder
- Himalayan salt to taste

Instructions:

1. Simply blend all the ingredients in a blender.
2. Add some Himalayan salt to taste.
3. Serve chilled, it's extremely refreshing and re-energizing.

Coconut milk and coconut oil make this recipe more nutritious (good fats!), so have no fear, they will not make you fat. In fact, coconut oil is recommended for weight loss and can also be used as a supplement. Personally, I consume about 2 tablespoons of coconut oil a day. It's a great wat to overcome sugar cravings in a healthier way.

Tofu and Spinach Curry

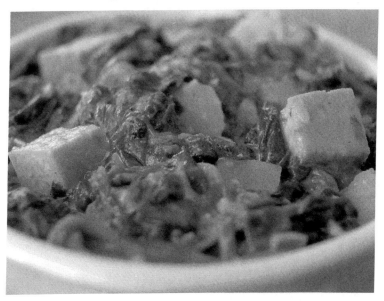

Ingredients:
- 1 cup diced tofu
- 2 cups chopped spinach
- 2 minced garlic cloves
- 1 medium onion, chopped
- 2 finely chopped tomatoes
- ½ cup coconut milk
- 1 bay leaf
- 1 teaspoon ginger
- ¾ teaspoon pepper
- ¾ teaspoon Himalayan salt
- ½ teaspoon turmeric powder
- coconut oil
- Some water

Method:

1. Heat some oil in a saucepan, sauté the garlic cloves and onion for about 3-4 minutes.
2. Add ginger, chopped tomatoes, turmeric powder, bay leaf and fry for another 3 minutes.
3. Throw in the spinach leaves, coconut milk, salt and cook until the spinach is slightly tender. Do not overcook the spinach.
4. Once this mixture cools down, blend it into a smooth paste.
5. Heat some coconut oil in another saucepan and shallow fry the tofu cubes until slightly golden brown.
6. Transfer the spinach curry in a sauce pan, add fried tofu and cook for 5-6 minutes with the lid covered.
7. Sprinkle some pepper on top and serve hot.
8. Enjoy!

Spinach, Kale and Tofu Pattie

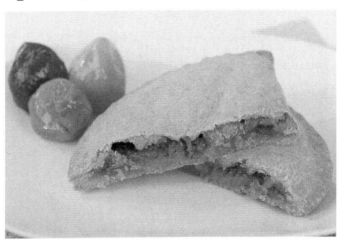

Serves: 3
Ingredients:

- ½ cup spinach
- ½ cup kale leaves
- 1 cup gluten free oats
- 1 medium onion, chopped
- 3 minced garlic cloves
- ½ cup tofu
- 1 teaspoon paprika powder
- ¾ teaspoon cayenne pepper
- cumin powder (1-2 teaspoons)
- ¾ teaspoon salt
- 4-5 tablespoons coconut oil
- Some water
- Some chopped coriander

Method:

1. Boil some water in a sauce pan, immerse the kale and spinach leaves for about 30 seconds and drain the water. Set aside.

2. Blend kale, spinach, oats, tofu, paprika, cayenne pepper, salt, cumin powder and onion.

3. Make small circular patties using your hands , set them aside

4. Heat some oil in a sauce pan.

5. Place all the patties onto it and shallow fry them for about 5-6 minutes on medium flame on both sides. Fry them until it turns golden brown.

6. Garnish with coriander on top.

Super Alkaline Soup

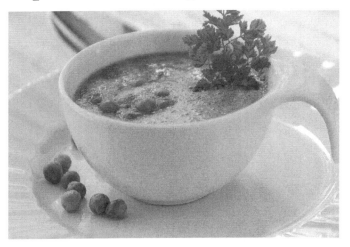

Serves: 2

Ingredients:

- 2 cups green peas
- 1 cucumber, peeled and chopped
- 1 chopped avocado
- 1 minced garlic clove
- 1 teaspoon minced ginger
- 2 cups vegetable broth
- ¾ teaspoon salt
- ½ teaspoon cayenne pepper
- Some mint sprigs
- 1 medium onion, chopped
- 1 tablespoon olive oil

Method:

1. Heat some olive oil in a sauce pan, sauté minced garlic, ginger and onion for about 2-3 minutes.

2. Add green peas, chopped avocado and sauté for 3-4 minutes until they are slightly tender.

3. Add the vegetable broth, cucumber, pepper, salt and

cook it for 3 minutes on medium flame.

4. Once this mixture cools down a slight bit, transfer it into a blender and blend until it forms a smooth paste. You can add some water if you want the soup to be thinner.
5. Refrigerate this soup for 2-3 hours.
6. Garnish with mint sprigs and/or other greens or vegetables of your choice and serve chilled on a hot sunny day.
7. Enjoy!

Asian Ginger Noodles

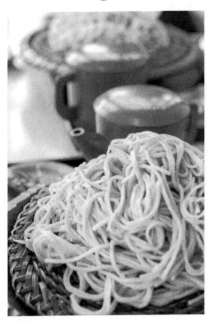

Serves: 3
Ingredients:

- 2 cups soba noodles
- 2 cucumbers, peeled and cut into thin strips
- ½ cup spinach leaves
- ½ cup kale leaves
- 1 medium onion, sliced
- powdered ginger (1 tablespoon)
- optional: soy sauce to taste (1-2 tablespoons)
- sesame oil or coconut oil (1-2 tablespoons)
- 2 tablespoons toasted sesame seeds
- 1 teaspoon red chili flakes
- ½ teaspoon pepper
- ¾ teaspoon salt
- 3 cups water to boil the noodles

- 1 tablespoon olive oil
- Some chopped cilantro

Method:

1. Take some water in a large sauce pan, add some olive oil and bring it to a boil.
2. Slide in the soba noodles, cook them for about 5-6 minutes until they are 75% cooked. Drain the water. Set aside.
3. Heat some sesame oil in a sauce pan, sauté the onions and garlic for about 3-4 minutes.
4. Add ginger, spinach, kale leaves, cucumber, soy sauce and cook for another 3 minutes.
5. Throw in the boiled soba noodles, add chili flakes, pepper, salt and fry for 2-3 minutes.
6. Garnish with some cilantro and serve hot.
7. Enjoy!

Ginger Cookies

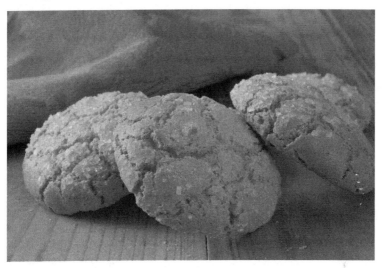

Ingredients:

- 1 cup coarsely ground almond flour
- ½ cup gluten-free oats
- ¼ cup coconut flour
- baking powder (1 teaspoon)
- cinnamon powder (1 tablespoon)
- ginger powder (1 tablespoon)
- ½ teaspoon all-spice powder
- ¼ teaspoon nutmeg powder
- 1 teaspoon vanilla essence
- 6-7 tablespoons coconut oil
- ¼ cup almond milk for binding

Method:

1. In a large bowl, combine almond flour, coconut flour, oats, baking powder, cinnamon, all spice powder, ginger, nutmeg powder and mix well.

2. Add vanilla essence, coconut oil, almond milk.

3. Set this mixture in the refrigerator for about 25-30 minutes until it becomes slightly firm.
4. Preheat the oven to 350°F.(180°C)
5. Split the cookie dough into 18-20 circular balls and place them on a baking sheet.
6. Bake the cookies for about 15 mins. Let them cool down.
7. Transfer them into an air-tight container and enjoy the cookies during breakfast or as an evening snack.
8. Enjoy!

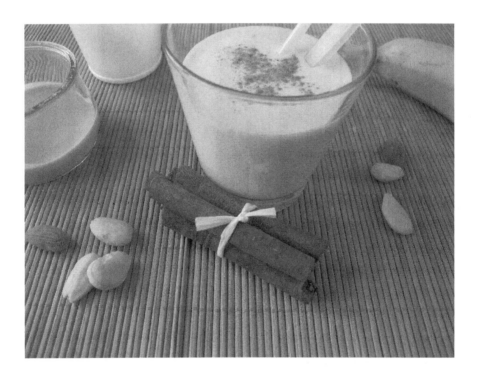

Beetroot Pudding

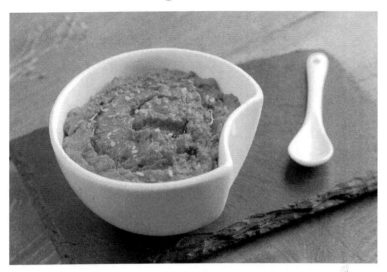

Do I love beets? Well, not really. Do I love this pudding? Yes!
Moreover this alkaline pudding helps me fight sugar cravings.
Try it yourself!

Serves: 3
Ingredients:

- 2 cups peeled and shredded beetroot
- 1 tablespoon coconut oil
- 2 tablespoons of almond butter
- 1 cup almond milk
- ¾ teaspoon cardamom powder
- ¼ teaspoon nutmeg powder
- 7-8 chopped almonds
- 7-8 chopped cashews
- ¼ cup raisins

Method:

1. Heat the coconut oil in a large sauce pan. Cook the shredded beetroot for about 12-15 minutes on low heat with the lid covered. Give it an occasional stir.

2. Add cardamom powder, almond milk and butter, nutmeg powder, raisins and cook for another 10-12 minutes on low heat. Remember to cover the saucepan with a lid. Stir occasionally.

3. Once the mixture cools down, refrigerate it for 60-90 minutes.

4. Heat another sauce pan and slightly roast the chopped almonds and cashews.

5. Garnish the beetroot pudding with toasted almonds and cashews on top.

6. Always serve chilled.

7. Enjoy!

Quinoa and Chickpea Curry

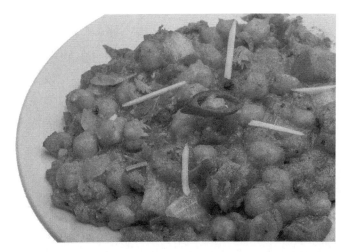

This one is really recommended if you want to show your friends that a vegan-alkaline diet is actually exciting and fun!

Serves: 2
Ingredients:
- 1 cup quinoa
- 1 cup chickpeas (soaked overnight)
- 1 minced garlic clove
- 1 teaspoon minced ginger
- 5-6 chopped spinach leaves
- 1 tablespoon lemon juice
- ½ cup diced sweet potato cubes
- 2 chopped tomatoes
- 1 medium onion, chopped
- 2 cups vegetable broth
- 1 teaspoon garam masala
- 1 bay leaf
- 1 teaspoon salt

- 2 tablespoon coconut oil
- Some cilantro for garnishing

Method:

1. Heat some oil in a sauce pan. Sauté the garlic and onion for about 3-4 minutes.
2. Throw in the bay leaves, spinach, chopped sweet potato, quinoa and cook for 5-6 minutes
3. Add the soaked chickpea, followed by some salt, garam masala and vegetable broth. Cook this curry for about 15-16 minutes on medium flame. Remember to cover the saucepan with a lid.
4. Sprinkle some lemon juice on top.
5. Garnish with some cilantro. So yummy and healthy!

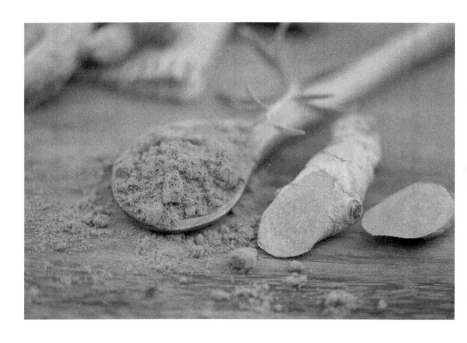

Spinach and Lemon Pesto

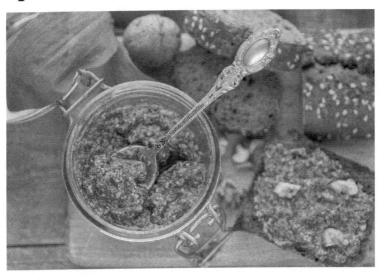

Serves: 4
Ingredients:

- 1 chopped avocado
- 1 cup spinach leaves
- 2 minced garlic cloves
- ½ teaspoon ginger
- Fresh juice of 2 big lemons
- ½ cup sliced shitake or button mushrooms (or any mushrooms of your choice)
- ½ cup cherry tomatoes
- 1 cup flat whole-wheat noodles (these are slightly acid-forming in the body, but OK occasionally, you can also use gluten-free noodles or skip this ingredient if you want it more alkaline)
- Himalaya salt (a pinch or two)
- pepper (up to 1 teaspoon)
- Some water to boil the noodles

- olive oil
- Some mint sprigs for garnish

Method:

1. Boil some water and add 1 teaspoon of olive oil.
2. Slide in the flat noodles and cook them for 5-6 minutes. Quickly drain the water. Set aside.
3. Place the spinach leaves, avocado and garlic along with very little water in a blender. Blend until smooth paste is achieved.
4. Heat some olive oil in a saucepan. Then sauté the mushrooms with cherry tomatoes.
5. Add the boiled noodles, followed by the spinach paste, salt, pepper and toss well.
6. Add some lemon juice.
7. Garnish with some mint sprigs and serve.
8. Enjoy!

Mexican Tortilla Soup

Even though this book is about Asian-Alkaline recipes, I couldn't resist and had to share this one. I hope you will enjoy it.

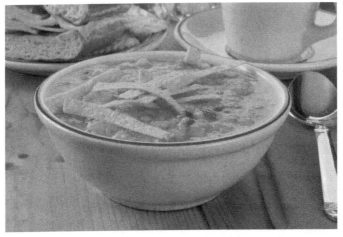

Serves: 2
Ingredients:
- 2 sprouted wheat wraps (gluten free "tortillas")
- 1 thinly sliced avocado
- 1 sliced red bell pepper
- 1 chopped tomato
- ½ cup spinach
- ½ cup sweet corn (small amounts of corn are fine as the rest of the ingredients will make this recipe more alkaline)
- 1 teaspoon soy sauce or garlic and herb infused olive oil (soy sauce is not alkaline)
- 2 minced garlic cloves
- ¾ teaspoon minced ginger
- Half jalapeno chili
- ¾ teaspoon Himalaya salt

- 1 tablespoon lemon juice
- 2 cups organic or home-made vegetable broth
- Some chopped parsley

Method:

1. Cut the tortilla sheet the way you want.
2. Take some vegetable broth along with some salt in a large sauce pan and bring it to a boil.
3. Add sliced avocado, bell pepper, spinach, corn, ginger, garlic, jalapeno chili, soy sauce and cook for about 10-12 minutes.
4. Slide in the tortilla strips and cook for another 4-5 minutes.
5. Drizzle some lemon juice on top.
6. Garnish with parsley or fresh cilantro (my fave!)
7. Serve with a few slices of lemon or lime. Enjoy!

Vegan Parsnip Super Alkaline Hummus

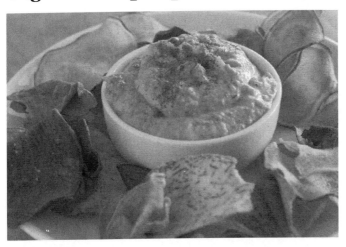

Who said that hummus is only about chickpeas? Let chickpeas have a break and try to be creative. All we need are alkaline veggies and spices....

Serves: 2

Ingredients:

- 4 chopped parsnips
- 2 smoked garlic cloves (or normal garlic)
- 2 tablespoons tahini
- 1 teaspoon cumin
- 2 tablespoons lemon juice
- ½ avocado
- Some mint sprigs
- 1 teaspoon Himalayan salt
- 2 cups water to boil parsnips
- ½ roasted bell pepper

- Some mint sprigs for garnish

Method:

1. Place some water in a large pot and bring it to a boil.

2. Slide in the chopped parsnips, avocado (don't boil if already soft- just add it in step 4) salt and boil for about 15 minutes until the ingredients turn tender. If you notice that the pieces are still firm, you can boil for another 6-7 minutes. Remember, the softer the parsnips and avocado, the smoother the dip will be.

3. Remove the excess water with a sieve and set aside to cool down.

4. Once cooled down, transfer this mixture to a food processor.

5. Add roasted garlic, bell pepper, salt, cumin, lemon juice to it and blend it until smooth.

6. Garnish the hummus with some mint sprigs and serve. I love it with quinoa or some raw veggies like carrots and cucumbers. It's also excellent for wraps.

7. Enjoy!

Baby Potato and Fenugreek Wraps

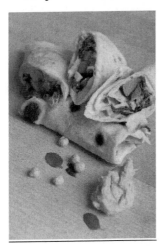

Serves: 3
Ingredients:
- 2 cups fenugreek leaves, thawed and chopped
- 1 cup baby potatoes
- 2 minced garlic cloves
- 1 finely chopped green chili
- 1 teaspoon coconut oil
- 1 teaspoon cumin
- 1 medium onion, chopped
- ¾ teaspoon salt
- 3 organic tortillas to make wraps (sprouted wheat wraps are my fave choice)
- Some water to boil potatoes

Method:
1. Boil the baby potatoes in some water for about 15-16 minutes until they are fully cooked. Once cooled down, peel them. Set them aside.
2. Heat some oil in a sauce pan; add cumin, minced garlic,

onion and sauté for about 3-4 minutes.

3. Add the chopped fenugreek, boiled potatoes, salt and cook for about 10-12 minutes with the lid covered.
4. Fill this mixture into each of the tortillas and serve.
5. Enjoy!

*** Fenugreek is an excellent source of Protein, Magnesium, Copper, Manganese, Dietary Fiber and Iron. It helps stimulate digestion, reduces inflammation and is recommended for weight loss.

Vanilla Flavored Quinoa Porridge

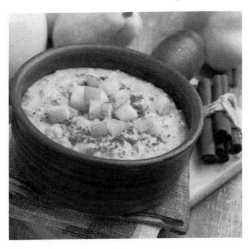

Serves: 3
Ingredients

- 1 cup quinoa
- 2 cups almond milk or coconut milk (don't count calories)
- 1 teaspoon vanilla essence or stevia (optional)
- ¼ cup chopped almonds
- ¼ teaspoon ground nutmeg
- ½ teaspoon cardamom powder
- 1 teaspoon freshly shredded ginger
- ¼ teaspoon salt

Method

1. Place some almond milk in a large vessel, add nutmeg powder, cardamom powder and bring it to a boil.
2. Add the quinoa; let it cook for about 12-15 minutes with the lid covered. Ensure that the quinoa is fully cooked.
3. Now throw in the shredded ginger, salt, vanilla essence, and let it simmer for about 7-8 minutes.

4. Once it cools down slightly, refrigerate this porridge for at least an hour before serving.

5. Heat a saucepan and slightly toast the chopped almonds on low heat.

6. Drizzle some over the quinoa porridge.

7. Serve slightly chilled (or nicely warm in the winter).

8. Enjoy! (I also like to add in some maca powder and cocoa for extra boost)

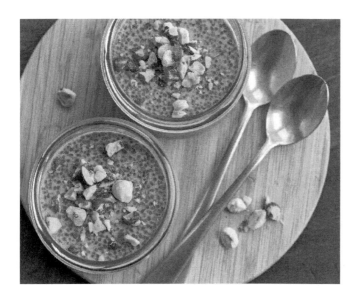

Spicy Thai Rolls

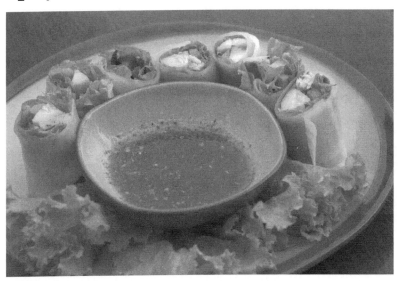

Serves: 4
Ingredients:

- 1 cup freshly shredded cabbage
- 1 cup freshly shredded carrot
- 1 sliced banana
- 8-10 chopped almonds
- 1 minced garlic clove
- 1 tablespoon sesame oil
- 1 tablespoons minced ginger
- 1 teaspoon chili flakes
- 2 teaspoons dried basil
- 10-12 Romanian lettuce leaves
- ¾ teaspoon Himalayan salt
- 1 tablespoon soy sauce or coconut oil infused with garlic and ginger (or both)
- 2 tablespoons soaked tamarind pulp
- 4 tablespoons pomegranate seeds

Method:

1. In a bowl, combine shredded carrot, cabbage, banana, ginger, garlic, pomegranate seeds, chili flakes, basil, tamarind pulp, soy sauce, sesame oil, salt and mix well. If you wish you can add some flax seeds to this mixture too.
2. Fill this mixture into each of the lettuce leaves gently and secure them with a toothpick.
3. Serve along with some mint sauce.
4. Enjoy!

Chickpea and Black Bean Salad

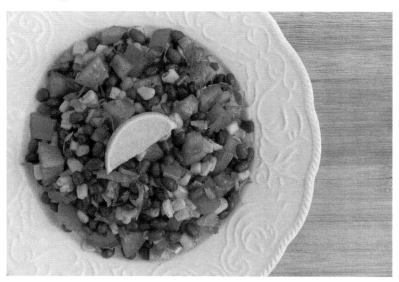

Serves: 4
Ingredients:
- ½ cup chickpea (soaked overnight)
- 1/2 cup black beans (soaked overnight)
- 2 cucumber, peeled and chopped
- 1 medium onion, finely chopped
- 1 chopped tomato
- 1 chopped raw mango
- 7-8 spinach leaves
- 1 teaspoon ground cumin
- 1 teaspoon raw mango powder
- 1/2 teaspoon Himalayan salt
- ¾ teaspoon cayenne pepper
- Some chopped cilantro
- Some water to boil the beans and chickpeas

Method:

1. Boil the chickpeas and black beans in about 3 cups of water. Drain and set aside.

2. Boil some water in another vessel and blanch the spinach for about 30 seconds. Drain the water.

3. In a large bowl, combine the chickpeas, blanched lettuce, cumin, chopped onion, chopped raw mango, dry mango powder, pepper, tomato, salt and mix well.

4. Garnish with some chopped cilantro and serve.

5. Enjoy!

Thai Green Curry

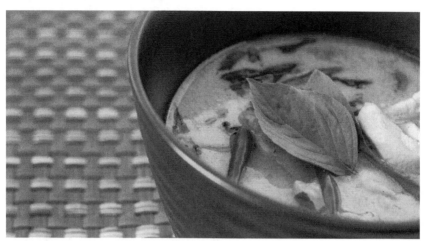

Serves: 3
Ingredients:

- ½ cup diced mushrooms
- 1 cup baby corns (GMO free)
- ½ cup chopped asparagus
- 1 chopped green bell pepper
- 1 medium onion, chopped
- 3 minced garlic cloves
- 1 chopped green chili
- 1 cup coconut milk
- 2 tablespoons Thai curry paste
- ¾ teaspoon salt
- ¾ teaspoon pepper
- 1 teaspoon dried basil
- 2 tablespoons coconut oil
- ½ cup vegetable broth

Method:

1. Heat some oil in a sauce pan. Sauté the onions and garlic for 3-4 minutes until the onions start to sweat.

2. Add the Thai curry paste. Then, pour the coconut milk slowly into the curry paste, followed by vegetable broth and bring it to a boil.

3. Add baby corns, asparagus, bell pepper, mushrooms, salt and cook for about 10-11 minutes.

4. Throw in the chopped green chili, basil leaves and give it a stir.

5. Serve alongside some brown rice.

6. Enjoy!

Quinoa and Bean Tacos

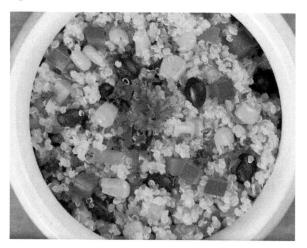

I always say that if you want to switch to an alkaline-vegan inspired lifestyle (even if you are not 100% vegan) quinoa should be one of the most important ingredients on your shopping list. There are hundreds of recipes that you can create with quinoa and it actually provides your body with natural, non-animal protein. Here comes another spicy alkaline recipe with quinoa.

Serves: 2
Ingredients:
- 1 chopped avocado
- 1 cup quinoa
- ½ cup black beans (soaked overnight)
- ½ cup sweet corn kernels
- ¾ teaspoon garlic powder
- 1 tablespoon lemon juice
- 2.5 cups vegetable broth
- 2 chopped tomatoes
- ½ teaspoon onion powder

- ¾ teaspoon salt
- 6-7 tortillas (alkaline friendly sprouted wheat wraps are the best)
- ½ teaspoon paprika powder
- Some chopped cilantro for garnish

Method:

1. Mix the quinoa in vegetable broth, boil it and cook for about 20 minutes.
2. Add the chopped tomatoes, black beans, garlic powder, onion powder, salt, corn kernels, paprika powder and cook again for about another 10-12 minutes. Keep the lid covered while cooking.
3. Sprinkle some lime juice on top and mix well.
4. Fill in this mixture into each of the tortillas and garnish with some cilantro.
5. Serve along with some barbecue sauce.
6. Enjoy!

Indian Smoked Egg Plant Curry

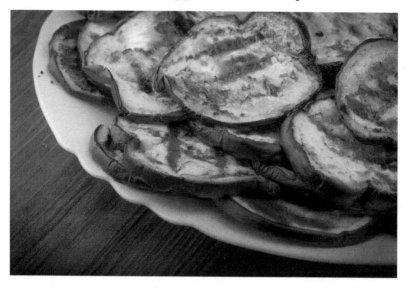

Serves: 3
Ingredients:

- 4 eggplants, sliced
- 1 tablespoons sesame oil
- 1 medium onion, finely chopped
- 3 minced garlic cloves
- 1 teaspoon minced ginger
- 1 slit green chili
- 2 tablespoons roasted groundnut powder
- 1 teaspoon mustard seeds
- ½ teaspoon cumin
- ¼ teaspoon asafetida
- ½ teaspoon turmeric powder
- 7-8 curry leaves
- Some chopped coriander leaves for garnish
- ¾ teaspoon salt

Method:

1. Coat the eggplant with a few drops of oil and rub it gently.

2. Now smoke them over a grill or medium flame from all sides for about 5-6 minutes. Ensure that the eggplant is properly smoked from all sides.

3. Once done, immerse them into a bowl full of chilled water. This helps in removing the skin faster. Once the skin is removed, mash them using a spatula or a spoon.

4. Heat some oil in a saucepan. Then add in the mustard seeds and cumin and let it crackle.

5. Add asafetida, green chili, turmeric, curry leaves, minced garlic, ginger and sauté for 2-3 minutes.

6. Add the chopped onion, tomatoes and fry them for 3 minutes. Switch off the flame

7. Transfer the mashed eggplant mixture to the saucepan, add some roasted groundnut powder, salt and mix well.

8. Garnish with some coriander leaves and serve.

9. Enjoy!

Steamed Vegetable Tofu Rolls

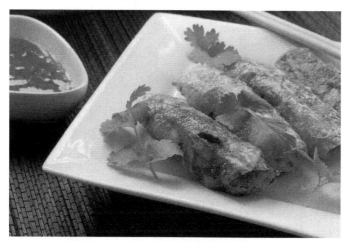

Tofu is another important ingredient for those who wish to embrace an alkaline-vegan lifestyle. It does not have to be boring to eat tofu. Preparing it and making it delicious and fun is actually an art. Let's dive into it!

Serves: 4
Ingredients:

- 2 cups shredded spinach leaves
- ½ cup bamboo shoots, thinly sliced into strips
- ½ cup chives, thinly sliced into strips
- 1 carrots, peeled and thinly sliced into strips
- 7-8 chopped spinach leaves
- ¼ cup sliced mushrooms
- 1 tablespoon soy sauce or olive oil infused with garlic and ginger
- 1 teaspoons freshly minced ginger
- 2 minced garlic cloves
- 100 ml water (0.4 cup)
- ½ cup tofu, mashed

- 1 teaspoon sesame oil
- ½ teaspoon pepper
- 1 chopped jalapeno chili
- 4 whole-wheat sheets or gluten free tortillas
- ¾ teaspoon Himalaya salt

Method:

1. Boil some water in a sauce pan and blanch the mushrooms for about 20 minutes. Drain the water and set aside.
2. Heat some oil in a saucepan, sauté the garlic, ginger, mushrooms, chives, bamboo shoots and carrots for about 5-6 minutes.
3. Add the spinach, jalapeño chili, salt, pepper, soy sauce, mashed tofu and stir fry them.
4. Once this mixture cools down, fill it gently into each of the tortillas and secure with a toothpick.
5. Serve along with some green salad.
6. Enjoy!

Lotus Root Soup

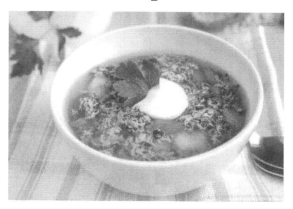

Serves: 3

Ingredients:

- 1 cup thinly sliced lotus roots
- 2 cups vegetable broth
- Some cilantro
- ½ cup chopped broccoli florets
- 1 minced garlic clove
- ½ teaspoon freshly shredded ginger
- ½ teaspoon salt
- 1 tablespoon lemon juice
- ½ teaspoon cayenne pepper
- 1 teaspoon olive oil

Method:

1. Heat some olive oil in a saucepan, sauté the garlic and shredded ginger for 2 minutes.
2. Throw in the lotus roots, broccoli and fry until they become slightly tender.
3. Add vegetable broth, lemon juice, salt, cilantro and cook the soup for about 15-16 minutes.
4. Sprinkle some pepper and serve along with some brown rice.

Squash and Carrot Curry

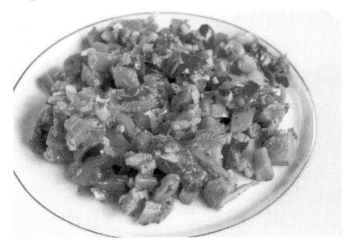

Serves: 2
Ingredients:

- 1 cup diced squash
- ½ cup diced carrots
- ½ cup chopped bell pepper
- 1/4 cup soy beans (make sure you use GMO free beans)
- 1 medium onion, chopped
- 3 minced garlic cloves
- 1 teaspoon minced ginger
- 1 red chili
- 1 teaspoon curry powder
- 1 teaspoon sesame oil
- 1 cup vegetable broth
- 1 bay leaf

Method:

1. Heat some oil in a sauce pan, sauté the ginger and garlic for 1-2 minutes.
2. Throw in the chopped onion, bay leaf, and fry until it turns golden brown.
3. Add red chili, soy beans, diced carrot, squash, bell

pepper, curry powder, vegetable broth and cook for 18-20 minutes with the lid covered.
4. Garnish with some chopped parsley on top and serve.
5. Enjoy!

Tasty Oats and Quinoa Pancakes

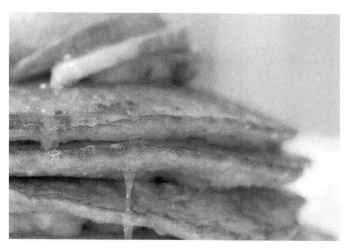

Serves: 3
Ingredients:
- ½ cup quinoa
- 1/4 oats
- 1 cup coconut milk or almond milk
- ½ cup freshly shaved coconut
- 1 tablespoon almond essence
- Coconut oil
- 1 tablespoon flax seeds
- ¼ teaspoon salt
- Some strawberry slices for garnish

Method:

1. In a food processor, grind the oats along with flax seeds, coconut and quinoa.
2. In a bowl, mix the ground coconut, flax seeds, quinoa, oats with almond milk, almond essence, salt and mix well. Set aside for 10 minutes.
3. Heat some almond oil in a saucepan; ensure that the oil is spread evenly across the pan.
4. Pour some pancake mixture onto the saucepan and cook for about 30-40 seconds from each side on medium heat.
5. Garnish the pancakes with some freshly chopped strawberry slices.
6. Enjoy!

Oyster Mushroom and Spaghetti Salad

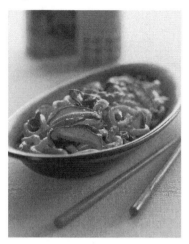

This is my slightly alkaline treat. Mushrooms and spaghetti are not alkalizing but you can have them every now and then (the alkaline diet allows you 30-20% of acid food in your diet). Remember to use organic ingredients and add plenty of green, alkaline foods as well as good oils (cold-pressed) to conjure up a balanced, slightly alkaline meal. Check it out and let me know what you (or your taste buds) think...

Serves: 3
Ingredients:
- 1 cup whole-wheat spaghetti (gluten free options are always more alkaline)
- 1 tablespoon sesame oil
- 1 minced garlic clove
- ½ teaspoon minced ginger
- 1 teaspoon caraway seeds
- ½ cup oyster mushrooms
- ¼ cup chopped kale leaves
- 1 tablespoon olive oil

- 1 chopped jalapeno pepper

- 1 tablespoon lemon juice
- Some chopped coriander
- 1 teaspoon salt
- ½ teaspoon pepper

Method:
1. Boil some water in a large vessel, throw in the spaghetti and cook for about 7-8 minutes. Drain the water and set aside.
2. In another sauce pan, take some olive oil, sauté the minced garlic, ginger, caraway seeds. This should take a few minutes.
3. Add the mushrooms, kale leaves, jalapeno chili, pepper, salt and stir fry for 3-4 minutes.
4. Once cooled down, transfer the mixture from the saucepan to a large bowl. Add the boiled noodles, sprinkle some lemon juice and toss well.
5. Garnish with some toasted sesame seeds and serve.
6. Enjoy!

Bok Choy Soup

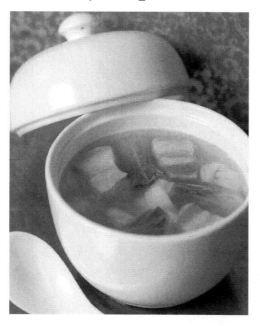

I know that the name of this recipe may sound weird to you, but don't get discouraged, this is an amazing soup that can warm you up in winter and take care of your immune system.

Ingredients:
Serves: 2

- 1.5 cup bok choy (white cabbage), thawed
- 4 minced garlic cloves
- 2 tablespoons olive oil
- 3 cups vegetable broth
- 2 tablespoons lemon juice
- ¾ teaspoon Himalayan salt
- ¼ teaspoons turmeric powder
- ½ teaspoon pepper powder

Method:

1. Heat some oil in a saucepan, sauté the garlic until it turn completely golden brown or starts giving a burnt smell.
2. Add some turmeric powder, bok choy, salt and sauté for 3-4 minutes.
3. Pour in the vegetable broth, lemon juice and let it simmer for a good 13-14 minutes. Stir occasionally while the soup is boiling.
4. Serve hot. Garnish with ground pepper.
5. Enjoy!

Optional: you can also use kale or spinach instead of bok choy

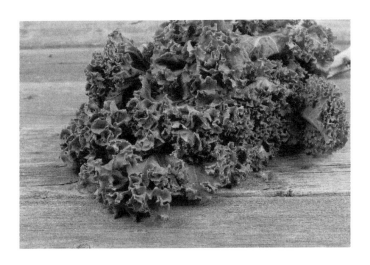

Thai Style Green Coconut Soup

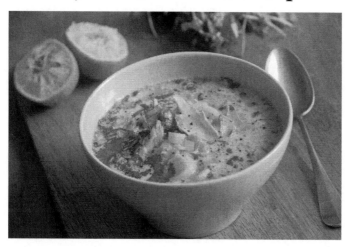

As a big fan of all coconut ingredients, I am naturally attracted to Thai cuisine. This soup can be served chilled or warm. I find it really refreshing and energizing especially after or before strenuous workouts.

Serves: 3
Ingredients:
- 1 cup freshly shaved coconut
- 2 cups coconut milk
- minced ginger (1-2 teaspoons, I like it hot so I go for more ginger)
- 1 minced garlic clove
- ½ teaspoon red chili flakes
- Coconut butter (1 tablespoon, I love it creamy!), if you can't get this ingredient, go for coconut oil or cream
- ½ teaspoon Himalayan salt
- 1 tablespoon lemon juice
- ¼ cup freshly chopped cilantro

Method:

1. Combine the shaved coconut, ginger, garlic, cilantro, coconut milk in a food processor and blend until smooth. Make sure not to leave any chunks.

2. Heat some coconut butter in a sauce pan; transfer the coconut puree into it.

3. Add some lemon juice and Himalayan salt. Simmer the mix for about 12- 15 minutes on low heat.

4. Garnish with some mint sprigs. Serve hot or chilled. If you are down with flu, this recipe is a natural, nourishing remedy that you should try.

5. Enjoy!

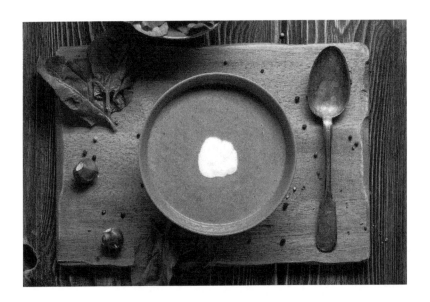

Stir Fry Eggplant

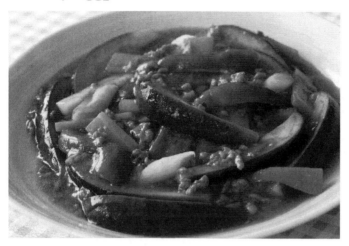

Serves: 2

Ingredients:

- 2 eggplants, sliced
- 1 medium onion, diced
- 3 minced garlic cloves
- 1 diced green bell pepper
- 1 diced red bell pepper
- 1 red chili
- 2 tablespoons olive oil
- 1 teaspoon dried basil
- 1 tablespoon of alkaline green powder or organic vegetable broth
- 2 tablespoons soy sauce
- ¼ cup water
- 1 teaspoon Himalaya salt

Method:

1. Heat some olive oil in a saucepan, sauté the minced garlic, red chili and diced onion for about 2 minutes.
2. Throw in the diced bell peppers, eggplants and stir fry for about 1-2 minutes.
3. Add soy sauce, dried basil, salt and stir fry it.
4. Mix one tablespoon of alkaline green powder with ¼ cup water.
5. Pour this liquid into the vegetable mixture and stir well. Cook for another 2-3 minutes until the mixture becomes thicker.
6. Sprinkle some black pepper and serve.
7. Enjoy!

Thai Red Curry

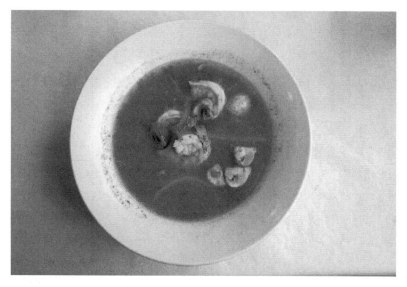

Here comes another amazing alkaline curry idea!

Serves: 4
Ingredients:
- 2 cups sweet potato, peeled and diced
- 2 carrots, peeled and diced
- 1/2 cup asparagus, peeled and diced
- 2 slit cayenne chilies
- ½ cup chopped dandelion greens
- 2 tablespoons Thai curry paste (vegan)
- 1 lime leaf
- 1 tablespoon dried basil
- ½ teaspoon salt
- 3 cups coconut milk
- Coconut oil

Method:

1. Heat the coconut milk in a large vessel and bring it to a boil.

2. Add the Thai curry paste to it, followed by diced sweet potatoes and let it cook for about 17-18 minutes until they are tender. Later add the lime leaf.

3. Heat some coconut oil in a saucepan; add asparagus, dandelion greens, dried basil carrots and stir fry them.
4. Transfer these sautéed veggies to the coconut mixture, add some salt and cook for another 2-3 minutes.
5. Garnish with some cayenne pepper and serve hot.
6. Enjoy!

Scrambled Tofu

I love this recipe for breakfast. It gives me all energy I need to be unstoppable throughout the day. Besides…I love the smells that it produces…it energizes me even further!

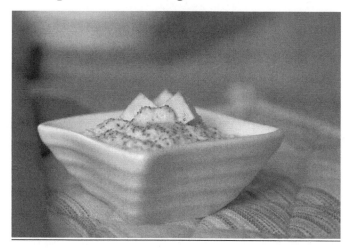

Serves: 2
Ingredients:

- 1 cup tofu
- 2 medium onions, diced
- 2 finely chopped tomatoes
- ½ cup green peas
- 1 teaspoon minced ginger
- 1 finely chopped green chili
- 1 bay leaf
- ¼ teaspoon garam masala
- 1 tablespoon coconut oil
- 1 tablespoon lemon juice
- ½ teaspoon black pepper
- ¾ teaspoon salt
- Some chopped coriander for garnish

Method:

1. In a bowl, crumble the tofu using your hands, set aside.
2. Heat some oil in a sauce pan, sauté the onions, bay leaf and garlic for 3-4 minutes on low heat.
3. Throw in the chopped tomatoes, green chili, green peas, cook for 3 minutes.
4. Add garam masala, salt and fry for another 1-2 minutes.
5. Sprinkle some lemon juice and pepper on top.
6. Garnish with some chopped coriander and serve along with some whole-wheat bread.
7. Enjoy!

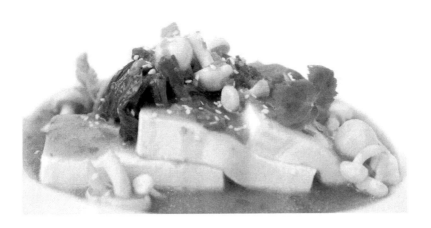

Stuffed Sweet Potato

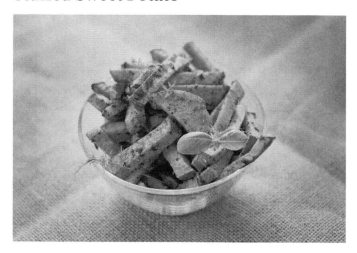

Serves: 3
Ingredients:

- 3 medium sweet potatoes
- 2 tablespoons coconut oil
- ½ cup chopped broccoli florets
- 3 diced tomatoes
- 1 finely chopped green bell pepper
- 1 teaspoon cumin
- Juice of 1 lemon
- Red chili flakes (1-2 teaspoons)
- 2 tablespoons dried dill leaves
- 2 minced garlic cloves
- ½ cup of soy sprouts
- ½ teaspoon Himalaya salt
- 1 teaspoon black pepper
- Some chopped parsley for garnish

Method:
1. Preheat the oven to 350°F. (180°C)
2. Wash the sweet potatoes properly and wipe them dry. Now slice them into two.
3. Coat the sweet potato slices with some coconut oil and set them on a baking tray. Bake it for 40-45 minutes until they are tender.
4. Once cooled down, scoop out the middle part and set them aside on a tray.
5. Heat the remaining coconut oil in a sauce pan, sauté the garlic, chopped broccoli florets, bell peppers, tomatoes for about 3-4 minutes.
6. Add sprouts, dried dill leaves, lemon juice, red chili flakes, salt and stir fry for another minutes. Switch off the flame.
7. Fill the veggie mixture into each one of the sweet potatoes carefully, sprinkle some pepper on top.
8. Garnish with some chopped parsley and serve.
9. Enjoy!

Tomato Curry

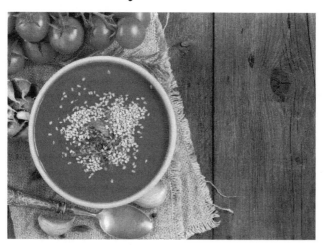

Serves: 2
Ingredients:

- 4-5 roughly chopped tomatoes
- 1-2 red chilies
- 8-10 curry leaves
- 1 medium onion, finely chopped
- 1/2 teaspoon mustard seeds
- ¼ teaspoon ground pepper
- 1 teaspoon cumin
- ¼ teaspoon turmeric powder
- ¼ teaspoon asafetida
- 2 teaspoons of coconut oil
- ½ teaspoon salt
- 1 cup coconut water (optional)
- Some chopped coriander leaves for garnish

Method:

1. Blend ripe tomatoes, onions in a blender and make a smooth lump-free paste. Strain it through a soup strainer to get a smooth tomato puree.
2. Heat some oil in a saucepan, throw in the mustard seeds, cumin and let them crackle.
3. Throw in the curry leaves, red chilies, asafetida, turmeric powder and sauté for 30-40 seconds.
4. Add the tomato puree to the saucepan, followed by some salt and cook for 3-4 minutes.
5. Add coconut water to get the desired consistency. Alternatively, you can also use alkaline water. Cook for another 5 minutes until the mixture thickens.
6. Sprinkle some ground pepper and garnish with some chopped coriander.
7. Enjoy!

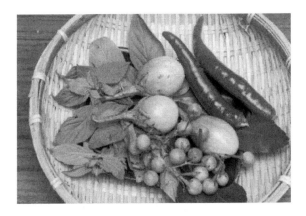

Spinach Garlic Absolute

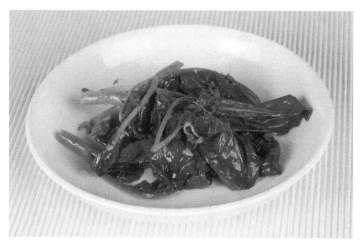

Ingredients:
Serves: 3

- 2 cups spinach leaves
- 6-7 minced garlic cloves
- 1 cup broccoli
- 2 boiled and diced potatoes
- 1 chopped zucchini
- 1 chopped carrot
- ½ cup soy beans , soaked as per instructions
- 1 teaspoon olive oil
- 2-3 cloves
- ½ teaspoon salt
- 1 cup vegetable broth
- 1 teaspoon pepper
- Some water to blanch spinach leaves

Method:

1. Boil some water and blanch spinach leaves in it for about one minute. Quickly run the blanched spinach through some chilled water. Doing this will retain its color.

2. Grind the blanched spinach along with some minced to make the basic sauce.

3. Heat some oil in a sauce pan, add some cloves, zucchini, carrot, soy beans and sauté for about 5-6 minutes until they turn slightly tender.

4. Add the pureed spinach, diced potatoes, salt, vegetable broth and cook for 12-13 minutes.

5. Sprinkle some ground pepper and serve along with some flat bread.

6. Enjoy!

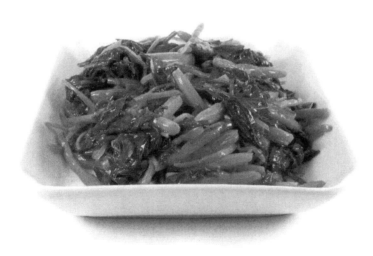

Yummy Quinoa Recipe

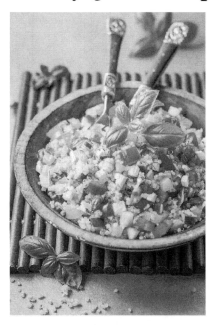

Serves: 2
Ingredients:

- 1 cup quinoa
- 2 onions, thinly sliced
- 1 bay leaf
- 2 whole cardamoms
- 2 cloves
- 1 teaspoon cumin
- 1 tablespoon ginger garlic paste
- 1 finely chopped tomato
- ½ teaspoon garam masala
- 2 slit green chilies
- 1 thinly sliced bell pepper
- 2 cups vegetable broth
- 8-9 chopped almonds

- 8-9 halved cashews
- ¼ cup raisins
- ¾ teaspoon salt
- 1 tablespoon coconut oil

Method:

1. Heat some oil in a sauce pan, throw in the cumin, green chilies, ginger-garlic paste, bay leaf, cardamoms, cloves and fry for 2-3 minutes.
2. Add chopped onions, tomatoes, bell pepper and sauté for 3 minutes.
3. Wash the quinoa, drain the water and transfer to the saucepan. Fry for 4-5 minutes on low heat.
4. Pour the vegetable broth, add some salt and cook for 18-20 minutes with the lid covered. Ensure that the quinoa is fully cooked.
5. Heat another sauce pan, slightly toast the almonds and cashews.
6. Garnish the pilaf with toasted nuts, raisins and serve hot.
7. Enjoy!

Banana and Sweet Potato Muffins

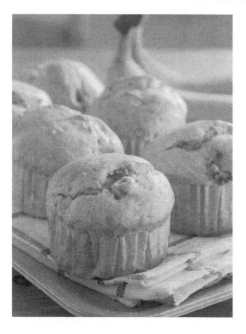

To be honest, this recipe is not really that alkaline (it's neutral) but it is one of my favorite homemade treats. It's still healthy and wholesome and can be a great step in the process of eliminating processed foods.

Serves: 2
Ingredients:
- 1 cup quinoa, cooked and dried
- ½ cup whole-wheat flour
- 1 teaspoon baking powder
- ½ teaspoon baking soda
- 1 tablespoons toasted flax seeds
- 2 ripe bananas, mashed
- 2 teaspoons vanilla essence
- 1 sweet potato, boiled and mashed
- ½ cup applesauce, unsweetened

- ½ teaspoon cinnamon
- ¼ teaspoon Himalaya salt

Method:

1. Preheat the oven to 390°F.(200 Celsius)
2. In a bowl, combine the quinoa along with flour, baking soda, baking powder, flax seeds and salt.
3. In another bowl, combine all the wet ingredients like mashed banana, mashed sweet potato and applesauce.
4. Transfer the wet ingredients to the dry ones and mix well using a beater.
5. Pour this batter into each muffin tin one by one.
6. Bake them for about 50 minutes to get fluffy and moist muffins.
7. Cool down in a fridge and enjoy! I love it with some homemade marmalade.

Lemon Flavored Zucchini Cream

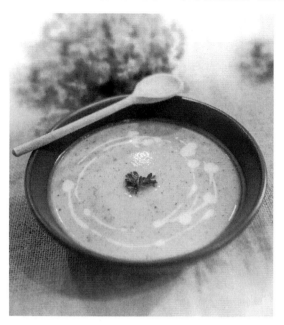

Serves: 2
Ingredients:

- 1 cup organic polenta
- 2 finely chopped zucchini
- 4-5 finely chopped kale leaves
- 1 tablespoon lemon juice
- Zest of two lemons
- ¼ cup mint sprigs
- 1 tablespoon olive oil
- ½ teaspoon pepper
- ½ teaspoon cumin powder
- 1 cup vegetable broth
- 1 teaspoon salt
- 1 teaspoon minced ginger
- Some chopped coriander

Method:

1. Heat some oil in a saucepan, sauté the minced ginger, cumin, kale leaves, chopped zucchini for about 3-4 minutes.

2. Add the polenta, lemon juice, lemon zest and fry for 4-5 minutes on medium heat.

3. Pour the vegetable broth in the saucepan, add some salt and cook for 14-15 minutes until the polenta is fully cooked.

4. Sprinkle some pepper, mix well.

5. Garnish with some chopped coriander and serve.

6. Enjoy!

Thai Alkaline Smoothie

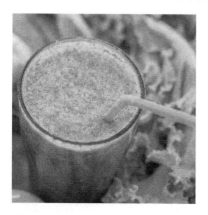

Serves: 2

Ingredients:

- 1 cup coconut water
- ¼ cup spinach leaves
- 1 cucumber, peeled and diced
- ¼ cup kale leaves
- 1 cup coconut cream
- Some fresh basil
- Some chopped coriander
- ¼ teaspoon salt
- 1 teaspoon lemon juice
- ¼ teaspoon pepper
- Some ice cubes

Method:

1. Wash the spinach leaves properly and put them in a grinder.
2. Add diced cucumber, coconut cream, chopped coriander, basil and blend it until smooth.
3. Add coconut water, salt, pepper and whisk again for about a minutes. Make sure it's nice and smooth.
4. Pour in a large glass, add some ice cubes and serve.

OPTIONAL: add some stevia or maple syrup to sweeten.

Garlic- Spinach Dal

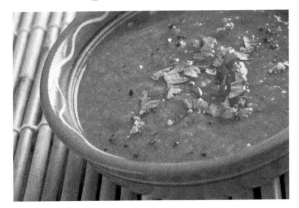

Serves: 2
Ingredients:

- 1 cup mung dal (soaked for 2 hours)
- 4 minced garlic cloves
- 1 teaspoon minced ginger
- 2 slit red chilies
- 1 teaspoon cumin
- 1 tablespoon sesame oil
- ½ cup chopped spinach
- 1 tablespoon lemon juice
- ½ teaspoon turmeric
- ¼ teaspoon asafetida
- 7-8 curry leaves
- 1 teaspoon salt
- 2 cups vegetable broth
- Some chopped coriander for garnish

Method:

1. Heat some oil in a large saucepan, throw in the mustard leaves, cumin, curry leaves and let them crackle.

2. Add turmeric powder, asafetida, red chilies, minced garlic, ginger and sauté for 1-2 minutes until the garlic

turn golden brown.

3. Add the chopped spinach leaves, soaked dal, salt, water and let it cook for 20-22 minutes on medium flame. Cover the lid while the dal is cooking.

4. Add some lemon juice, sprinkle some chopped coriander and serve.

5. Enjoy!

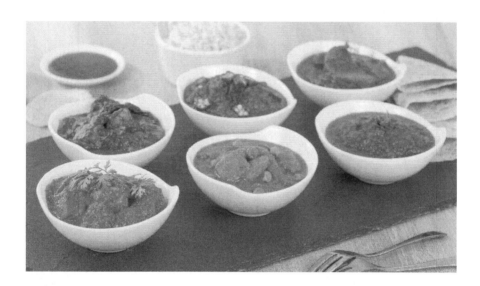

Peach Neutral Smoothie

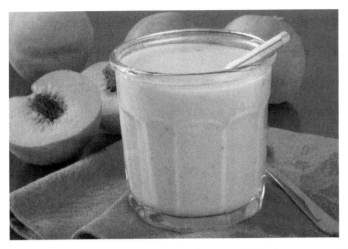

This mildly alkaline/neutral smoothie is a naturally sweet treat that will help you eliminate processed sweets from your diet.

Serves: 2

Ingredients:

- 2-3 ripe peaches, diced
- ½ teaspoon cardamom powder
- Half banana, chopped
- ¼ cup lemon juice
- 2 cups almond milk
- 1 teaspoon chia seeds
- Some ice cubes

Method:

1. Combine the diced peaches, banana, almond milk and orange juice in a food processor and blend until smooth.
2. Sprinkle some cardamom powder and stir it well.
3. Pour the smoothie into large glasses.
4. Add some ice cubes and enjoy!

Couscous with Lentils

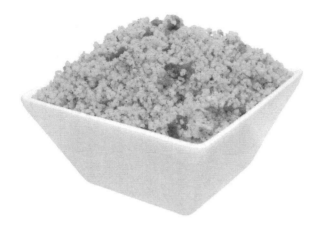

This recipe is simple, healthy, balanced and easy to prepare. Make sure you go for gluten-free couscous. It's great as a warm-up dish for long, cold winter evenings.

Serves: 2

Ingredients:

- 1 cup tomato juice (homemade, simply blend a few tomatoes, no peel)
- ½ cup vegetable broth
- 3 minced garlic cloves
- Olive oil (1 tablespoon)
- 1/2 cup lentils, cooked
- 3 diced tomatoes
- 1 cup couscous, soaked in water
- ½ teaspoon Himalayan salt
- 1 teaspoon ground pepper
- Coconut oil (1 tablespoon)

Method:

1. Heat some oil in a saucepan, sauté the garlic until it turns slightly golden.
2. Throw in the chopped tomatoes; stir fry for 3-4 minutes.
3. Add couscous, lentils, vegetable broth, tomato juice, salt and cook for about 5 minutes on a low flame so that lentils and couscous take a nice taste.
4. Sprinkle some black pepper, add more salt if you wish and serve.
5. Enjoy!

Simple Broccoli Detox Soup

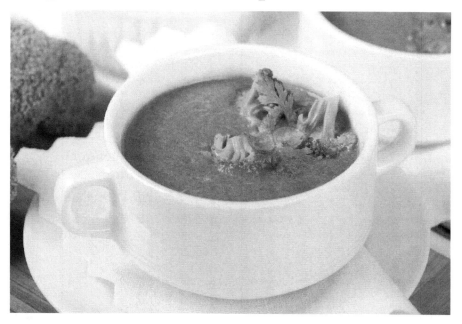

Serves: 2

Ingredients:

- 2 cups broccoli florets
- 2 garlic cloves
- 2 big carrots
- 2 cups of water
- 1 cup coconut milk
- 1 cup almond milk
- Himalaya salt
- Spicy pepper powder
- Curry powder
- Olive oil
- Rings of 1 onion, fried (optional)

Method:

1. Put some water (about 2 cups) to boil and add carrots, garlic and broccoli.

2. Turn of the heat when boiling. Add a bit of olive oil and Himalaya salt. Cover the pot and let the veggies cool down.

3. When cooled, blend all the ingredients.

4. Add some almond milk and coconut milk to make it more or less creamy depending on your preferences. Add more water if you do not want it too thick.

5. Spice it up with curry and pepper. I also like to throw in some lentils or quinoa if I need more quick energy.

6. Re-heat slightly or served chilled. I love to add some fried onions to give it more taste, but this is up to you.

7. Enjoy! This is a really powerful detox!

Simple Exotic- Alkaline Refreshing Juice

Lemons and grapefruits, even though acidic fruits at first glance and acidic in taste, actually have an alkalizing effect on your body once metabolized. Yes! They are low in sugar and high in minerals and vitamins which makes them alkaline-forming, detoxifying fruits. If for whatever reason you can't stand them because of their acidic taste, try to use them to infuse water or mix with other fruits. Like I said at the beginning of this book - the most important thing is to listen to your body.

This recipe uses natural stevia to sweeten and the juices are diluted in almond and coconut milk which makes it easier for newbies. Coconut water is miraculous and great for refreshment and alkalization.

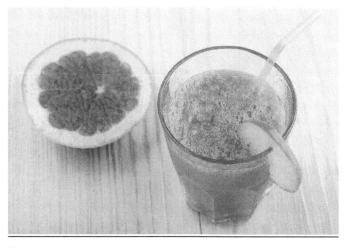

Serves: 2
Ingredients:
- Juice of 4 grapefruits
- Juice of 2 lemons
- 1 cup coconut water
- 1 cup coconut milk

- 1 cup almond milk
- 1 tablespoon of ginger powder
- OPTIONAL: stevia to sweeten
- OPTIONAL: 1 tablespoon of green, alkaline powder (for example barley grass)

Method:
Simply mix all the ingredients and add some ice cubes.
Garnish your glass with a slice of lemon or lime. Enjoy! I love this juice before and after my workouts.

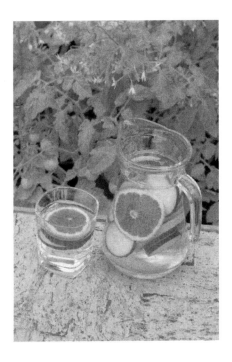

Oriental Summer Salad Recipe

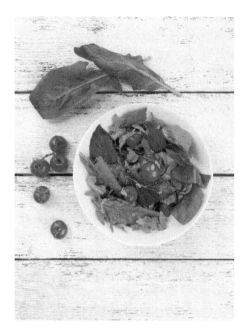

This recipe is really quick to prepare and will help you energize your body and mind. It offers oriental taste, refreshment and pH balancing properties.

Serves: 2
Ingredients:
1 avocado, peeled, pitted and sliced
2 big tomatoes
2 garlic cloves, minced
1 cup arugula leaves
¼ cup cilantro
1 cucumber, peeled and sliced
Half an apple, peeled and sliced
½ cup of basmati rice, cooked and cooled
¼ cup almonds
Himalayan salt
Juice of 1 lemon

¼ cup coconut milk
½ teaspoon curry powder

Method:
Place all the salad ingredients in a bowl and stir well.
Mix lemon juice with coconut oil, Himalayan salt and curry
powder.
Spread the salsa over the salad.
Enjoy!

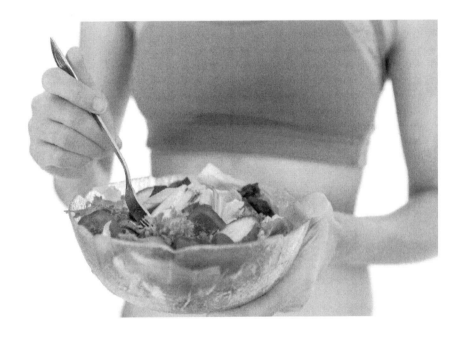

BONUS CHAPTER

EXOTIC SMOOTHIE RECIPES

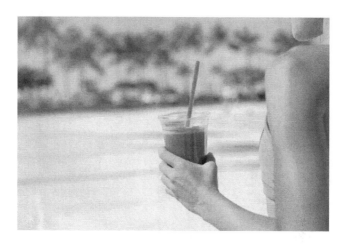

Rhubarb and Avocado Satisfying Smoothie

Serves: 2
Ingredients:
2 cups rhubarb
2 avocados
2 cups coconut water
2 tablespoons lemon juice
1 cup almond milk, raw
1 tablespoon coconut oil
1 teaspoon cinnamon

Instructions:
Clean and place the rhubarb in boiling water. Leave for 5 minutes. Drain and set aside.
Meanwhile, deseed the avocado and scoop out the flesh.
Place the avocado flesh in blender. Add coconut water, almond milk and rhubarb.
Blend until smooth.

Add in the lemon juice, cinnamon and coconut milk.
Place it in a glass and serve. Garnish with a slice of lemon.
Enjoy!

Spicy Creamy Smoothie

Serves: 2
Ingredients:
2 cups coconut flesh
2 cups coconut cream
2 tablespoons cinnamon powder
1 tablespoon clove powder
1 teaspoon cayenne pepper
1 teaspoon ginger powder
1 teaspoon garlic powder
1 teaspoon cumin powder
1 teaspoon coriander powder
A pinch of Himalayan crystal salt

Instructions:
Place the coconut flesh and coconut water in a blender and
blend until fully smooth and creamy.
Heat all of the spices on a very low flame for 10 minutes. Keep
a close eye on these. Place the coconut mix in a glass and stir
in 2 tablespoons of the spice mix into it.
Sprinkle some salt on top and serve chilled.
Enjoy!

Basil Coconut Smoothie

Serves: 2-4
Ingredients:
2 cups fresh basil leaves
2 cups fresh mint leaves
2 cups almond milk
1 cup coconut water
1 cup coconut cream
2 tablespoons flax seed oil
2 tablespoons coconut oil
2 tablespoons cilantro leaves
Ice cubes

Instructions:
Thoroughly cleanse the basil and mint leaves and place in boiling water for 2 minutes. Strain, but set water aside.
Place the almond milk and coconut cream in a blender and blend until completely smooth.
Place the leaves in a blender along with the coconut water and blend until smooth.
Add the coconut flesh, flax seed oil, and ice cubes to the blender. Blend until smooth.
Mix this with the mint water and coconut oil. Place it in a glass.
Serve with some fresh cilantro on top.
Enjoy!

Wheat Grass and Papaya Smoothie

Serves: 4
Ingredients:
½ cup wheat grass, juiced
2 teaspoons sea kelp powder (optional)
2 cups coconut water
2 tablespoons Udo's oil
2 tablespoons dates
A few pineapple slices (optional)
2 cups of papaya slices
Cinnamon
Ice cubes

Instructions:
Place the dates in boiling water and allow it to soften completely.
Juice wheat grass and set aside. Wheat grass can be also used directly in a smoothie, but I prefer to juice it and then add it to my smoothie (it's easier to digest juiced).
Chop the dates and papaya.
Blend the coconut water, dates, pineapple, papaya and Udo's oil until creamy.
Add wheat grass juice, kelp powder and mix again.
Pour it into a tall glass and sprinkle some cinnamon and nutmeg powder on top. Enjoy!

CONCLUSION

So, how was your experience? Have you tried any of my recipes yet? If not, make sure you start by preparing a shopping list and setting a date for your own healthy dinner party. This can be an amazing opportunity for you to socialize, save up money (restaurants can be expensive), learn new skills, and spread the word of wellness. Alcohol is off of the alkaline diet, as it is acid forming. However, you can treat yourself to a couple of glasses of good organic wine over the weekend, this can be a really nice addition to your alkaline dinner. Remember - wine is less acidic than beer or spirits. Additionally, make sure you drink plenty of good quality, filtered water to remain hydrated. Hydration and alkalinity go hand in hand.

Finally, I would like to encourage you to carry on your research on the alkaline diet. There are many ways you can practice this diet, ranging from the more radical alkaline approach (it consists of eating only alkaline foods and is normally recommended for those who were doing a Standard Western Diet for a really long time) to a balanced alkaline diet (this is the approach I use). Everyone is different. If you want to learn holistic nutrition you must learn to listen to your body first.

In reducing processed foods from your diet, you are working to prevent many potential diseases such as cancer, diabetes, arthritis and many more. On top of that, you are providing your family with important nutritional foundation that they need to create a life full of happiness, energy and fulfilment.

If you enjoyed my book, it would be greatly appreciated if you left a review so others can receive the same benefits you have. Your review can help other people take this important step to take care of their health and inspire them to start a new chapter in their lives.

At the same time, <u>you can help me serve you and all my other readers</u> even more.

I'd be thrilled to hear from you. I would love to know your top 3 recipes.

Simply visit the link below or go <u>to your Amazon orders and write a short review</u> to share your experience. I know you are busy and I would like to thank you in advance for considering taking a couple of minutes to review this book.

Link (amazon US): <u>www.amazon.com/author/mtuchowska</u>

Honestly, whenever I get a review, I jump around like a little kid and I read it all over again, my cheeks rosy with excitement!

You can also reach me via email:
<u>info@holisticwellnessproject.com</u>

Have a fantastic day,

I wish you all the best on your journey

Marta Tuchowska

<u>www.HolisticWellnessProject.com</u>

<u>www.AlkalineDietLifestyle.com</u>

ADDITIONAL RESOURCES FOR ALKALINE WELLNESS MOTIVATION

Looking for more recipes and wellness?

Follow me on Instagram and discover my holistic lifestyle secrets + dozens of alkaline recipes, picks and motivational videos that will help you keep on track throughout the day:

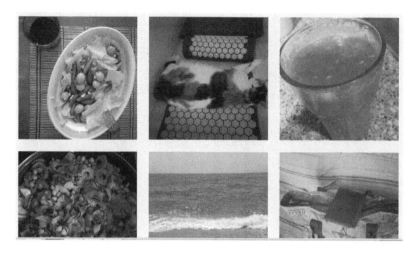

www.instagram.com/Marta_Wellness

Free eBook

Don't forget to download your free copy of "Revolutionize Your Life with Alkaline Foods"

Download Link:
www.holisticwellnessproject.com/alkaline

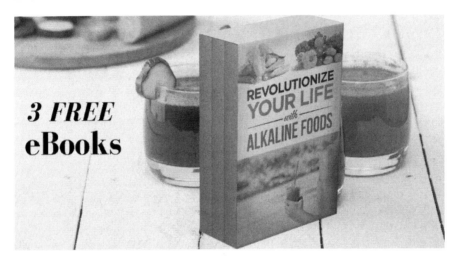

More Wellness Books by Marta Tuchowska (available in all Amazon stores, simply search for "Marta Tuchowska") or visit:

www.holisticwellnessproject.com/alkaline-diet-books

www.amazon.com/author/mtuchowska

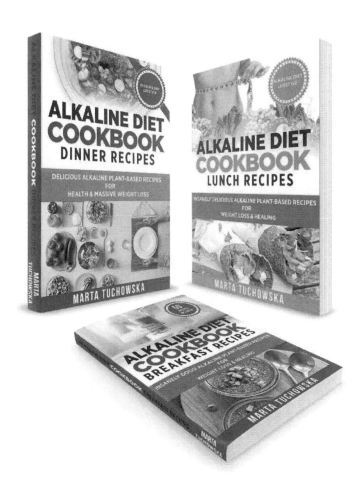